MY DOG
JOURNAL

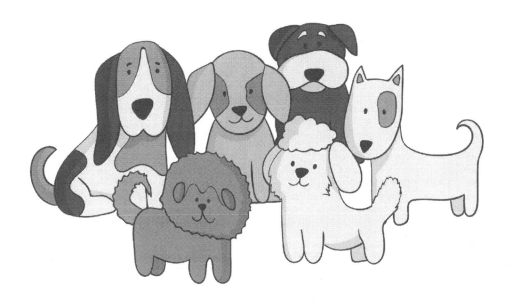

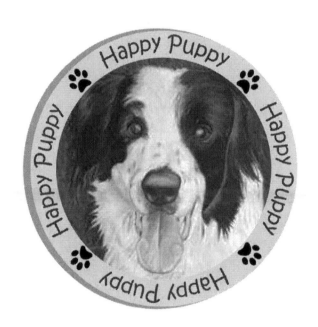

HAPPY PUPPY PLANET

Written With Love By:

_____

_____

_____

If found, please return to me

My Dog's Story

PHOTO

Write about meeting your dog for the first time. Where did you find him? Did you meet his parents? Why did you choose this dog?

THE TEN BEST THINGS
ABOUT MY DOG

1. _____

2. _____

3. _____

4. _____

5. _____

6. _____

7. _____

8. _____

9. _____

10. _____

woof 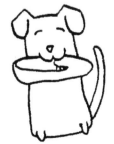 woof

MY DOG'S PROFILE

NAME _____

NICKNAME _____

ADOPTION DATE _____

SHELTER/BREEDER _____

BREED _____

GENDER _____

SPAYED/NEUTERED _____

LICENSE #, STATE _____

COLOR _____

EYE COLOR _____

RABIES TAG # _____

INSURANCE INFORMATION

    COMPANY _____

    POLICY # _____

    PHONE/WEBSITE _____

MICROCHIP

    COMPANY _____

    CHIP # _____

    PHONE _____

PERSONALITY _____

FEARS _____

MY DOG'S FAVORITES

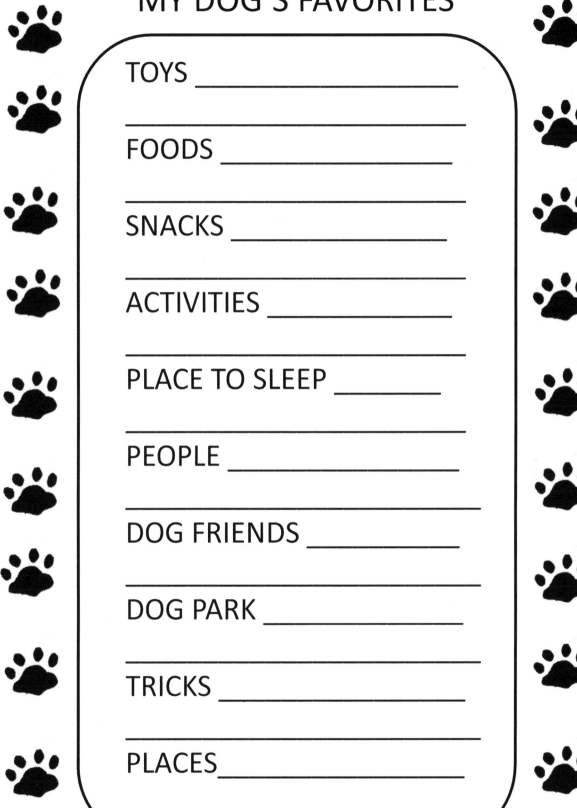

TOYS _____

_____

FOODS _____

_____

SNACKS _____

_____

ACTIVITIES _____

_____

PLACE TO SLEEP _____

_____

PEOPLE _____

_____

DOG FRIENDS _____

_____

DOG PARK _____

_____

TRICKS _____

_____

PLACES_____

_____

VET VISITS

DATE	REASON	DIAGNOSIS	TREATMENT	COST

VET VISITS

DATE	REASON	DIAGNOSIS	TREATMENT	COST

VET VISITS

DATE	REASON	DIAGNOSIS	TREATMENT	COST

VET VISITS

DATE	REASON	DIAGNOSIS	TREATMENT	COST

VACCINATION CHART

DATE	TYPE	VET	INJECTION SITE	NEXT DUE DATE	NOTES

VACCINATION CHART

DATE	TYPE	VET	INJECTION SITE	NEXT DUE DATE	NOTES

VACCINATION CHART

DATE	TYPE	VET	INJECTION SITE	NEXT DUE DATE	NOTES

VACCINATION CHART

DATE	TYPE	VET	INJECTION SITE	NEXT DUE DATE	NOTES

MEDICAL CONDITIONS

DATE	VET	CONDITION	TREATMENT	PROCEDURE	INJURIES

MEDICAL CONDITIONS

DATE	VET	CONDITION	TREATMENT	PROCEDURE	INJURIES

MEDICATION TRACKER

MED	VET	REASON	DOSE & FREQUENCY	METHOD	START DATE	END DATE

MEDICATION TRACKER

MED	VET	REASON	DOSE & FREQUENCY	METHOD	START DATE	END DATE

MEDICATION TRACKER

MED	VET	REASON	DOSE & FREQUENCY	METHOD	START DATE	END DATE

MEDICATION TRACKER

MED	VET	REASON	DOSE & FREQUENCY	METHOD	START DATE	END DATE

EXPENSES

DATE	TYPE (VET, FOOD, TOYS, GROOMER, ETC)	COST

EXPENSES

DATE	TYPE (VET, FOOD, TOYS, GROOMER, ETC)	COST

EXPENSES

DATE	TYPE (VET, FOOD, TOYS, GROOMER, ETC)	COST

EXPENSES

DATE	TYPE (VET, FOOD, TOYS, GROOMER, ETC)	COST

TRAINING

COMMAND: _____
START DATE: _____LEARNED _____

COMMAND: _____
START DATE: _____LEARNED _____

COMMAND: _____
START DATE: _____LEARNED _____

COMMAND: _____
START DATE: _____LEARNED _____

COMMAND: _____
START DATE: _____LEARNED _____

COMMAND: _____
START DATE: _____LEARNED _____

FAVORITE TRAINING INCENTIVES:

☐ CLICKER   ☐ PRAISE

☐ FOOD

IMPORTANT PHONE NUMBERS

VET
NAME
ADDRESS
PHONE

EMERGENCY VET
NAME
ADDRESS
PHONE

PETSITTER
NAME
ADDRESS
PHONE

GROOMER
NAME
ADDRESS
PHONE

KENNEL
NAME
ADDRESS
PHONE

POISON CONTROL
PHONE

PET SITTER NOTES

VISITS PER DAY _____

FOOD_____

WATER _____

WALKS _____

VET NAME & PHONE _____

FAVORITE GAMES _____

FAVORITE TOYS _____

WHERE TO FIND
    FOOD _____
    LEASH _____
    MEDICATIONS _____
    POOP BAGS _____

MEDICATIONS
    DOSE _____
    HOW TO GIVE _____
    WHEN TO GIVE _____

SPECIAL INSTRUCTIONS _____

My Dog's Story

PHOTO

Write about meeting your dog for the first time. Where did you find him? Did you meet his parents? Why did you choose this dog?

THE TEN BEST THINGS
ABOUT MY DOG

1. _____

2. _____

3. _____

4. _____

5. _____

6. _____

7. _____

8. _____

9. _____

10._____

woof 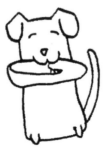 woof

MY DOG'S PROFILE

NAME _____

NICKNAME _____

ADOPTION DATE _____

SHELTER/BREEDER _____

BREED _____

GENDER _____

SPAYED/NEUTERED _____

LICENSE #, STATE _____

COLOR _____

EYE COLOR _____

RABIES TAG # _____

INSURANCE INFORMATION

    COMPANY _____

    POLICY # _____

    PHONE/WEBSITE _____

MICROCHIP

    COMPANY _____

    CHIP # _____

    PHONE _____

PERSONALITY _____

FEARS _____

MY DOG'S FAVORITES

TOYS _____

_____

FOODS _____

_____

SNACKS _____

_____

ACTIVITIES _____

_____

PLACE TO SLEEP _____

_____

PEOPLE _____

_____

DOG FRIENDS _____

_____

DOG PARK _____

_____

TRICKS _____

_____

PLACES_____

_____

VET VISITS

DATE	REASON	DIAGNOSIS	TREATMENT	COST

VET VISITS

DATE	REASON	DIAGNOSIS	TREATMENT	COST

VET VISITS

DATE	REASON	DIAGNOSIS	TREATMENT	COST

VET VISITS

DATE	REASON	DIAGNOSIS	TREATMENT	COST

VACCINATION CHART

DATE	TYPE	VET	INJECTION SITE	NEXT DUE DATE	NOTES

VACCINATION CHART

DATE	TYPE	VET	INJECTION SITE	NEXT DUE DATE	NOTES

VACCINATION CHART

DATE	TYPE	VET	INJECTION SITE	NEXT DUE DATE	NOTES

VACCINATION CHART

DATE	TYPE	VET	INJECTION SITE	NEXT DUE DATE	NOTES

MEDICAL CONDITIONS

DATE	VET	CONDITION	TREATMENT	PROCEDURE	INJURIES

MEDICAL CONDITIONS

DATE	VET	CONDITION	TREATMENT	PROCEDURE	INJURIES

MEDICATION TRACKER

MED	VET	REASON	DOSE & FREQUENCY	METHOD	START DATE	END DATE

MEDICATION TRACKER

MED	VET	REASON	DOSE & FREQUENCY	METHOD	START DATE	END DATE

MEDICATION TRACKER

MED	VET	REASON	DOSE & FREQUENCY	METHOD	START DATE	END DATE

MEDICATION TRACKER

MED	VET	REASON	DOSE & FREQUENCY	METHOD	START DATE	END DATE

EXPENSES

DATE	TYPE (VET, FOOD, TOYS, GROOMER, ETC)	COST

EXPENSES

DATE	TYPE (VET, FOOD, TOYS, GROOMER, ETC)	COST

EXPENSES

DATE	TYPE (VET, FOOD, TOYS, GROOMER, ETC)	COST

EXPENSES

DATE	TYPE (VET, FOOD, TOYS, GROOMER, ETC)	COST

TRAINING

COMMAND: _____
START DATE: _____LEARNED _____

COMMAND: _____
START DATE: _____LEARNED _____

COMMAND: _____
START DATE: _____LEARNED _____

COMMAND: _____
START DATE: _____LEARNED _____

COMMAND: _____
START DATE: _____LEARNED _____

COMMAND: _____
START DATE: _____LEARNED _____

FAVORITE TRAINING INCENTIVES:
- [ ] CLICKER   [ ] PRAISE
- [ ] FOOD

IMPORTANT PHONE NUMBERS

VET
NAME
ADDRESS
PHONE

EMERGENCY VET
NAME
ADDRESS
PHONE

PETSITTER
NAME
ADDRESS
PHONE

GROOMER
NAME
ADDRESS
PHONE

KENNEL
NAME
ADDRESS
PHONE

POISON CONTROL
PHONE

PET SITTER NOTES

VISITS PER DAY _____

FOOD_____

WATER _____

WALKS _____

VET NAME & PHONE _____

FAVORITE GAMES _____

FAVORITE TOYS _____

WHERE TO FIND
    FOOD _____
    LEASH _____
    MEDICATIONS _____
    POOP BAGS _____

MEDICATIONS
    DOSE _____
    HOW TO GIVE _____
    WHEN TO GIVE _____

SPECIAL INSTRUCTIONS _____

My Dog's Story

PHOTO

Write about meeting your dog for the first time. Where did you find him? Did you meet his parents? Why did you choose this dog?

THE TEN BEST THINGS
ABOUT MY DOG

1. _____

2. _____

3. _____

4. _____

5. _____

6. _____

7. _____

8. _____

9. _____

10. _____

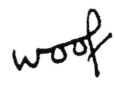 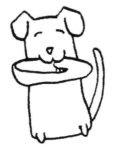 woof   woof

MY DOG'S PROFILE

NAME _____

NICKNAME _____

ADOPTION DATE _____

SHELTER/BREEDER _____

BREED _____

GENDER _____

SPAYED/NEUTERED _____

LICENSE #, STATE _____

COLOR _____

EYE COLOR _____

RABIES TAG # _____

INSURANCE INFORMATION

    COMPANY _____

    POLICY # _____

    PHONE/WEBSITE _____

MICROCHIP

    COMPANY _____

    CHIP # _____

    PHONE _____

PERSONALITY _____

FEARS _____

MY DOG'S FAVORITES

TOYS _____

_____

FOODS _____

_____

SNACKS _____

_____

ACTIVITIES _____

_____

PLACE TO SLEEP _____

_____

PEOPLE _____

_____

DOG FRIENDS _____

_____

DOG PARK _____

_____

TRICKS _____

_____

PLACES_____

_____

VET VISITS

DATE	REASON	DIAGNOSIS	TREATMENT	COST

VET VISITS

DATE	REASON	DIAGNOSIS	TREATMENT	COST

VET VISITS

DATE	REASON	DIAGNOSIS	TREATMENT	COST

VET VISITS

DATE	REASON	DIAGNOSIS	TREATMENT	COST

VACCINATION CHART

DATE	TYPE	VET	INJECTION SITE	NEXT DUE DATE	NOTES

VACCINATION CHART

DATE	TYPE	VET	INJECTION SITE	NEXT DUE DATE	NOTES

VACCINATION CHART

DATE	TYPE	VET	INJECTION SITE	NEXT DUE DATE	NOTES

VACCINATION CHART

DATE	TYPE	VET	INJECTION SITE	NEXT DUE DATE	NOTES

MEDICAL CONDITIONS

DATE	VET	CONDITION	TREATMENT	PROCEDURE	INJURIES

MEDICAL CONDITIONS

DATE	VET	CONDITION	TREATMENT	PROCEDURE	INJURIES

MEDICATION TRACKER

MED	VET	REASON	DOSE & FREQUENCY	METHOD	START DATE	END DATE

MEDICATION TRACKER

MED	VET	REASON	DOSE & FREQUENCY	METHOD	START DATE	END DATE

MEDICATION TRACKER

MED	VET	REASON	DOSE & FREQUENCY	METHOD	START DATE	END DATE

MEDICATION TRACKER

MED	VET	REASON	DOSE & FREQUENCY	METHOD	START DATE	END DATE

EXPENSES

DATE	TYPE (VET, FOOD, TOYS, GROOMER, ETC)	COST

EXPENSES

DATE	TYPE (VET, FOOD, TOYS, GROOMER, ETC)	COST

EXPENSES

DATE	TYPE (VET, FOOD, TOYS, GROOMER, ETC)	COST

EXPENSES

DATE	TYPE (VET, FOOD, TOYS, GROOMER, ETC)	COST

TRAINING

COMMAND: _____
START DATE: _____LEARNED _____

COMMAND: _____
START DATE: _____LEARNED _____

COMMAND: _____
START DATE: _____LEARNED _____

COMMAND: _____
START DATE: _____LEARNED _____

COMMAND: _____
START DATE: _____LEARNED _____

COMMAND: _____
START DATE: _____LEARNED _____

FAVORITE TRAINING INCENTIVES:

☐ CLICKER   ☐ PRAISE

☐ FOOD

IMPORTANT PHONE NUMBERS

VET
NAME
ADDRESS
PHONE

EMERGENCY VET
NAME
ADDRESS
PHONE

PETSITTER
NAME
ADDRESS
PHONE

GROOMER
NAME
ADDRESS
PHONE

KENNEL
NAME
ADDRESS
PHONE

POISON CONTROL
PHONE

PET SITTER NOTES

VISITS PER DAY _____

FOOD_____

WATER _____

WALKS _____

VET NAME & PHONE _____

FAVORITE GAMES _____

FAVORITE TOYS _____

WHERE TO FIND
    FOOD _____
    LEASH _____
    MEDICATIONS _____
    POOP BAGS _____

MEDICATIONS
    DOSE _____
    HOW TO GIVE _____
    WHEN TO GIVE _____

SPECIAL INSTRUCTIONS _____

Made in the USA
Middletown, DE
29 August 2022

72543595R00066